T0271516

TEACHING EMPATHY AND CONFLICT RESOLUTION TO PEOPLE WITH DEMENTIA

of related interest

Adaptive Interaction and Dementia
How to Communicate without Speech
Dr Maggie Ellis and Professor Arlene Astell
Illustrated by Suzanne Scott
ISBN 978 1 78592 197 1
eISBN 978 1 78450 471 7

**Understanding Behaviour in Dementia
that Challenges, Second Edition**
A Guide to Assessment and Treatment
Ian Andrew James and Louisa Jackman
ISBN 978 1 78592 264 0
eISBN 978 1 78450 551 6

Embracing Touch in Dementia Care
A Person-Centred Approach to Touch and Relationships
Luke Tanner
Foreword by Danuta Lipinska
ISBN 978 1 78592 109 4
eISBN 978 1 78450 373 4

Positive Communication
Activities to Reduce Isolation and Improve the Wellbeing of Older Adults
Robin Dynes
ISBN 978 1 78592 181 0
eISBN 978 1 78450 449 6

Positive Psychology Approaches to Dementia
Edited by Chris Clarke and Emma Wolverson
Foreword by Christine Bryden
ISBN 978 1 84905 610 6
eISBN 978 1 78450 077 1

Person-Centred Dementia Care, Second Edition
Making Services Better with the VIPS Framework
Dawn Brooker and Isabelle Latham
ISBN 978 1 84905 666 3
eISBN 978 1 78450 170 9

TEACHING EMPATHY AND CONFLICT RESOLUTION TO PEOPLE WITH DEMENTIA

A Guide for PERSON-CENTERED PRACTICE

CAMERON CAMP AND LINDA CAMP

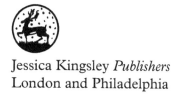

Jessica Kingsley *Publishers*
London and Philadelphia

Poem on pp.12-13 reprinted with kind permission of Naomi Drew.

First published in 2018
by Jessica Kingsley Publishers
73 Collier Street
London N1 9BE, UK
and
400 Market Street, Suite 400
Philadelphia, PA 19106, USA

www.jkp.com

Library of Congress Cataloging in Publication Data
Names: Camp, Cameron J., author. | Camp, Linda, 1952- author.
Title: Teaching empathy and conflict resolution to people with dementia : a
   guide for person-centred practice / Cameron Camp and Linda Camp.
Description: London ; Philadelphia : Jessica Kingsley Publishers, 2018. |
   Includes bibliographical references.
Identifiers: LCCN 2017036917| ISBN 9781785927881 (alk. paper) | ISBN
   9781784507374 (eISBN)
Subjects: | MESH: Dementia--rehabilitation | Negotiating--methods | Empathy |
   Person-Centered Therapy--methods
Classification: LCC RC521 | NLM WM 220 | DDC 616.8/31--dc23 LC record
available at https://lccn.loc.gov/2017036917

British Library Cataloguing in Publication Data
A CIP catalogue record for this book is available from the British Library

ISBN 978 1 78592 788 1
eISBN 978 1 78450 737 4

Printed and bound by CPI Group (UK) Ltd, Croydon, CR0 4YY

CONTENTS

THE RESULT OF SUCCESS

We are witnessing a quiet revolution in dementia care. It involves the emergence of an emphasis on seeing the *person* in the "person with dementia." It can be found in the use of terms such as "person-centered care" or "person-focused care" (Mast, Shouse and Camp 2015). It is seen in the development of "Dementia Friendly Communities" in Europe, Australia, Asia, and North America. These developments reflect a shift in focus. We are witnessing the advent of a new paradigm, in which we see dementia as a disability rather than a disease per se. We are viewing individuals with dementia as persons rather than as patients.

One aspect of this revolution is the development of the model of dementia care that reflects the role of a person with dementia within a community. In residential care, this means creating communities of persons with dementia living together, who are in turn connected with the larger community and the world. If successful, we shall see groups of individuals living together who feel free to express their preferences as they always have done. They will expect their preferences to continue to be given due attention and respect, and sometimes will differ in their opinions with one another. In other words, as in any community, you will have disagreements and disputes, some of which may be emotionally charged. This will be the inevitable result of this revolution if it is successful.

You do not see many disputes among rows of "patients" sitting in chairs or wheelchairs who do not converse or engage with the world. These people are easy to control, but they are not truly living. It is not the way we would want to live. The model of dementia care we create today is the one we will live in ourselves. We must be prepared to deal with the result of a successful revolution. That is the focus of this book, and the reason it has been written.

We wish to thank Melanie Tusick, who was instrumental in helping us bring this work to completion. We thank Michelle Lee, Ph.D., Miriam Rose, and Ross Wilkoff, who provided feedback on earlier drafts of this book. We thank our colleagues in other countries, especially Jerome Erkes and Veronique Durand, for their support and ideas. We also thank the students, family members, residents, and staff members we have worked with over the years for the opportunity to learn from them.

Cameron and Linda Camp
Solon, OH, USA
May, 2017

CHAPTER 1

MODELING PEACE AND EMPATHY

THEY WILL LEARN FROM WATCHING YOU

We begin this book with a simple idea—to teach persons how to handle conflict and feel empathy for others, we must demonstrate these abilities ourselves. If we tell others not to shout and then lose our tempers and shout at others, our words and lessons are meaningless. Especially as dementia advances, persons reflect the environment around them. They will take their cue on how to act, what to feel, etc. by looking at our faces, hearing our voices, and reflecting back what they see in us. And so, we begin with a journey inward.

There are three key values that underlie our approach—respect, dignity, and equality—based on our experience translating the work of Maria Montessori into dementia care. We assume that these three values should guide all interactions among humans—that any person should be treated with respect, with dignity, and as our equal. How do these values manifest themselves in behavior that we can, in turn, model for others? Here are some examples:

- We do not call another person names or disparage their ideas.

- We do not raise our voices when having a discussion or conflict.

- We acknowledge that we will have "good" days and "bad" days, but that we cannot use this as an excuse for treating others badly.

- We say a "Pledge of Peace" at the start of each day, to remind ourselves of what is truly important and, if possible, we make this a part of the routine for the persons with dementia we work with and care for. Places to find examples of peace pledges are found in Appendix 1.

- We treat other persons the way we wish to be treated.

- We work hard at listening to other people and try to understand their thoughts and feelings.

- We communicate our empathy and understanding of others' thoughts and feelings.

- We recognize that persons who are different from us and who have different life experience also have worth and that we can learn from these persons.

- We treat everyone we meet with respect, dignity, and equality—especially those persons with whom we disagree or whom we do not particularly enjoy being with.

- We literally and figuratively do not talk down to, or talk over, other persons. (We speak face-to-face at the eye level of a person we are addressing. We do not shout or communicate to other persons who are some distance away while standing next to a person with dementia. We do not speak about a person who is present as if the person was not present.)

- We realize that persons, especially those with dementia, must learn to trust us and that we must earn their trust.

- We work to develop and maintain healthy, affirming relationships.

- We promote harmony rather than dissension, cooperation rather than conflict.

Here is an example of a "Montessori Pledge" that is useful to remember at the start of the day when working in a residential setting for persons with dementia:

I will:

- work to create a place where I would want to live.

- remember that I am a guest in the home of my residents.

- remember that I must earn the trust of others, and that they must learn to trust me.

- treat everyone I encounter with respect, dignity, and equality.

- remember to treat others the way I wish to be treated.

(Center for Applied Research in Dementia (n.d.))

Persons with dementia (and without dementia) will learn about peace and empathy through our example. In Chapter 6, we discuss teaching mindfulness to persons with dementia. This can only be successful if we practice mindfulness ourselves, which includes a commitment to daily meditation.

It will soon become obvious that this book is not just about how to enable persons with dementia to resolve conflicts. This is a manifesto regarding how we should live our lives as civilized, caring human beings. We make the assumptions that life is not a zero-sum game, that we should treat others the way we wish to be treated, and that individuals with dementia have the capacity to learn, create new habits, and develop new abilities and beliefs—including those required to live peacefully and productively. Our mission is to enable all of us to join together on this journey to a better life. Here is a poem that exemplifies these ideas:

IT STARTS WITH YOU
by Naomi Drew

Let the eyes
inside your heart
see into the hearts
of others.

Realize
they have the need
to be accepted
just like you.

Let them see you care,
open up your mind,
treat them with respect,
show that you're a friend.

When you do this
you might find
others treating
you the same,

opening their eyes
to look inside your heart
returning the respect
you have given them.

And one by one
the world may change;
a brighter sun
might start to rise,

reminding us
that peace for all
is rooted in
the things we do.

(Drew 1999, p.2)

With these thoughts in mind, let us begin.

CHAPTER 2

WHAT IS PEACE?

A DEFINITION OF PEACE

1. a state of tranquility or quiet: such as

   a. freedom from civil disturbance

   b. a state of security or order within a community provided for by law or custom

2. freedom from disquieting or oppressive thoughts or emotions

3. harmony in personal relations

   a. a state or period of mutual concord between governments

   b. a pact or agreement to end hostilities between those who have been at war or in a state of enmity

"Peace" adapted from Merriam-Webster.com (2017)

All aspects of this definition of peace should relate directly to person-centered care for individuals with dementia. It is their (and our) right to live in a place that is tranquil (in the sense of not producing anxiety) and secure—a place where these states of being are sustained by a set of codes or customs created and maintained by persons with dementia and those who provide care to them. Thus, social and physical environments must enable individuals with dementia to be free from disquieting or oppressive thoughts or emotions. Additionally, these environments must promote concord as well as a means of resolving disagreements among persons with dementia and those who provide their care.

Peace, therefore, involves a process whereby persons take care of themselves, of each other, and of their social and physical environments. This is true of all persons, with or without dementia. The challenge to bringing peace to dementia care is threefold. First, how can we enable this process to be successful in spite of the cognitive challenges of persons with dementia? Second, how can we circumvent physical challenges associated with geriatric populations that often co-occur in populations with dementia? And finally, how can we enable this process to be successful in settings where individuals who have not lived together before and/or who have lived together under different circumstances must interact?

Imagine a university dormitory setting in which students arrive for their first year of study. Many have not lived away from home before. There are disparate personalities, social classes, habits and customs, and even primary languages. Somehow this group of individuals must coalesce into a group that can function as a community and live harmoniously. This does not occur at once, but if there are clear rules of conduct enforced by persons with authority who also can model appropriate behaviors, a (relatively) peaceful dormitory community can emerge.

Now imagine a classroom with 24 preschool students aged three to five years. They arrive on the first day of school, many not wishing to be there. The role of their teacher (often called a "guide" in Montessori classrooms) is to enable these very individual children to socialize, and to help these children interact, share, and resolve conflicts. Their teacher will do this through modeling, role playing, and enabling the students to practice peaceful behaviors. In addition, exercises will be presented regularly to enable the development of empathy for others. Like the university students, some of these children will not have had extensive practice inhibiting impulses, sharing, tolerating opinions that differ from theirs, dealing with external authority, or accepting limitations on what they can do. They must learn, at least within the confines of their classroom and school, to work within a system that is designed to produce cooperation and harmony rather than hedonism.

Finally, imagine a dementia care residence such as an assisted living community that is just opening. Twenty-four older adults with dementia, many not wishing to be there, arrive over the course of a few months and now are expected to live together. There are disparate personalities, social classes, habits and customs, and even primary languages. They must learn to interact, share, and resolve conflicts. Many residents have not had recent experience or practice inhibiting impulses, sharing, tolerating opinions that are different from theirs, accepting limitations on what they can do, etc. Somehow, they must coalesce into a group that can function as a community and be able to live harmoniously. Further, this must be done in spite of an array of cognitive and physical challenges common in this population.

> *True peace, on the contrary, suggests the triumph of justice and love among men; it reveals the existence of a better world wherein harmony reigns.*
>
> (Montessori 1971, p.7)

The point of these scenarios is that creating and maintaining peace among persons with dementia has many parallels to other life scenarios, and as a result we can utilize knowledge and techniques from a wide variety of sources when working with persons with dementia. In addition, we must be cognizant of the unique attributes of persons with dementia and adapt approaches to peace to meet the needs of this population. While this is our challenge, it also is our hope. We do not need to create an approach "from scratch," and we can utilize our knowledge of dementia to guide our development of peaceful living environments for these persons.

HOW DO WE BEGIN TO CREATE A PEACEFUL AND PEACE-PROMOTING ENVIRONMENT FOR PERSONS WITH DEMENTIA?

First, we must come to recognize that these issues are much larger than policies involving how to provide residential care for persons with dementia. They touch upon universal beliefs about the rights of human beings and the values that should support human beings. To illustrate this, let us examine some text from the United Nations' Universal Declaration of Human Rights.[1]

---

1   www.un.org/en/udhrbook/pdf/udhr_booklet_en_web.pdf

Article 1

All human beings are born free and equal in dignity and rights. They are endowed with reason and conscience and should act towards one another in a spirit of brotherhood.

Article 3

Everyone has the right to life, liberty and security of person.

Article 29

1. Everyone has duties to the community in which alone the free and full development of his personality is possible.

2. In the exercise of his rights and freedoms, everyone shall be subject only to such limitations as are determined by law solely for the purpose of securing due recognition and respect for the rights and freedoms of others and of meeting the just requirements of morality, public order and the general welfare in a democratic society.

Article 30

Nothing in this Declaration may be interpreted as implying for any State, group or person any right to engage in any activity or to perform any act aimed at the destruction of any of the rights and freedoms set forth herein.

So, the question is, does the system of residential dementia care as currently practiced in most of the world support or deny these basic human rights? It is interesting that the typical mission and values statements of residential care settings for persons with dementia usually reflect universal beliefs about the rights of human beings and the values that should support human beings. But an objective assessment of the current state of dementia care, as generally practiced, would provide a negative answer to the question in most instances.

When we are in France, providing training in the creation of resident-led communities in dementia care to staff members of long-term care residences, we find it useful to bring up the national motto—three words that we see throughout France on buildings, banners, etc. In English, the words are: Liberty, Equality, and Fraternity. At that point, we ask a very basic question: Should these rights be surrendered when a person is given the diagnosis of dementia?

CHAPTER 3

WORKING WITH PERSONS WITH DEMENTIA

What are the differences between working with persons with dementia and working with other groups? The primary difference, in many instances, involves the pattern of cognitive deficits that identify the condition known as dementia. One challenge involves difficulty remembering recent events or conversations. This can make it difficult for persons with dementia to remember conversations about resolving conflicts, instances where the person may have insulted or behaved aggressively towards another individual, and other elements involved with learning peaceful behaviors, conflict resolution, etc. They also may have difficulty inhibiting or controlling emotional outbursts, as well as difficulty expressing their thoughts clearly.

In addition, dementia is most commonly seen in older adults, who also may have a variety of physical challenges and medical conditions, such as problems with mobility, decreased strength, high blood pressure, diabetes, incontinence, poor vision and/or hearing, complications from taking multiple medications, etc. These, acting in combination with the cognitive deficits associated with dementia, serve as challenges in creating a peaceful and conflict-free environment for persons with dementia. With the additional effects of coming to live in a residential setting that may be unfamiliar to them, with people who are unfamiliar to them, and being placed in such a setting against their will, it is not surprising that many dementia care environments are far from peaceful.

Imagine the following scenario in a memory care unit for persons with dementia. Two residents become agitated with one another. One (a woman) insults the other (a man), and swings her walker at him, grazing his arm. The man says "I don't have to take this from anyone!" and storms back to his room. Both residents continue to feel upset. A staff member comes to the woman and says, "You should apologize to Mr. _____. What you did was not very nice." The woman, still angry, turns on the staff member and says, "What are you talking about? I didn't do anything to anyone! Leave me alone, you (insert curse word here)." Another staff member goes to the man in his room and says, "You seem upset, Mr. _____. Is there anything I can do?" The man, still agitated and angry, turns on the staff member and shouts, "Get out of here and leave me alone!"

Let us examine how this might come about. Two persons who have difficulty remembering recent events have an argument, and then have difficulty remembering the details of the argument. Imagine if you are told that you did something wrong and you cannot remember doing it. What would your reaction be? Usually, you would deny that you had done it, and you might well be angry at your (unjust) accuser. We also know that strong emotions can linger or resonate for some time after an event (this is true for persons with or without dementia). And so, you might be feeling upset or angry for no apparent reason when your accuser confronts you. What would you do or say? As Maya Angelou said, "I've learned that people will forget what you said, people will forget what you did, but people will never forget how you made them feel." The point to be made is that the persons in the above scenario are acting as you would act. They are acting normally, given the circumstances. This is why it is so important to understand how dementia does and does not influence conflicts and our attempts to train conflict resolution.

HOW COULD WE ADDRESS THIS CONFLICT BETWEEN THIS MAN AND WOMAN?

The best way for dealing with the situation above is to prevent it from happening in the first place. This begins by knowing the persons with dementia in our care, not just their names and disabilities, but who they are as persons. Of course, conflicts inevitably will arise when people live together. When conflicts do arise, there are ways to actively deal with a tense situation, as we discuss in Chapter 5. Here, we will discuss our ultimate goals: to enable persons with dementia to develop habits that will lead to a reduction or absence of conflict, or will enable them to manage conflict themselves.

First, contrary to what you might have read elsewhere, persons with dementia have the capacity to learn far into the course of dementia. Learning and memory have different components and are dependent on different parts of the brain. Learning systems that are acquired early in life tend to be retained far into the course of dementia. These include the learning of locations, habits, categorizing, motor learning, improvement with practice, and conditioning (both classical and operant) (Camp 2006a, 2012, 2013; Camp and Nassar 2003; Camp and Skrajner 2016; van der Ploeg *et al.* 2013).

When we train them, we ask staff members the following question: "Imagine that you are bringing residents of a dementia residential unit to eat lunch, and you notice that some resident already has taken the chair that is 'Henry's' chair. When Henry comes to the dining room, what will happen?" At this point, most persons in the room groan. They know that Henry will be upset that someone has taken "his" chair. Then we say, "If Henry came here because of a diagnosis of dementia, and *after* he came here he *learned* that this was his chair for lunch, he has shown the ability to continue learning after receiving a diagnosis of dementia."

Persons with dementia are learning on a regular basis, but we have not been encouraged or trained to see and use this capacity. The forms of learning available to persons with dementia generally involve learning that is unconscious, automatic, and effortless. You do not consciously think about the chair you normally sit in when you eat lunch, you simply sit there once, remember the location, sit there again, and form the habit of sitting in "your" place. This is a "learning by doing" system. It is our responsibility to guide persons with dementia into doing behaviors that will enable good habits (such as how to resolve conflicts and how to experience empathy) to be formed.

THE PREEMPTIVE NICE

Imagine a resident with dementia who acts in a very hostile way towards a staff member assigned to provide personal care to the resident. Many times, staff members may come from a different cultural or racial background than the resident, which may lead to the resident using insults and racial slurs against the staff member. Here is an example of a training exercise for staff members that we refer to as a "preemptive nice."

The staff member providing care to the hostile resident has been told not to "take it personally" because "it is the disease that is talking." Being human, that is very hard to do, especially when you must encounter this daily. The staff member learns to avoid this resident as much as possible, only coming near when personal care must be provided, and saying little or nothing as a way of "being patient" while verbal and sometimes physical abuse is inflicted by the resident. Of course, if this resident gets the reputation of being a "problem" resident, other staff begin to stay away as well. As a result, the resident's main social interactions with other humans may only occur when the resident is being abusive. So the cycle builds on itself and is perpetuated. There must be a different way to deal with this situation.

Why is this happening? In addition to the challenges of dementia mentioned earlier, we also may have to deal with old habits such as prejudice. How can we help the resident and staff member so that new habits and ways of interaction can replace the old ones? The preemptive nice is one approach to this. It takes advantage of an element of classical conditioning—the conditioned emotional response. We wish to create a new association—a positive feeling in the "challenging" resident towards the staff member. This can be done by continuously pairing the presence of the staff member with a positive emotion in the resident.

We say to the staff member, "When you begin and end your shift each day, spend 30 seconds or so doing this exercise. Approach the resident (staying at arm's length) and say something nice, such as 'I really like your sweater' or 'I'm so glad to see you up and out of your room.' After that you can walk away. This will be a very different episode and occurrence than what this resident usually experiences. If the resident says something negative, ignore it. If the resident says or does anything positive, reflect it back, such as by saying, 'I see a smile on your face. You really are beautiful when you smile.'"

This is about creating a new association in the person with dementia. The resident can, with repetition, begin to experience positive feelings toward the staff member. The resident may not remember these episodes, but their effects begin to accumulate. In other words, the resident can learn to like the staff member. It does not matter if the resident does not know why this positive feeling is there. This also occurs because the staff member has formed a new habit. In addition, the staff member can learn to like the resident, because classical conditioning is a form of learning seen in persons with or without dementia.

It also is important to do and say the same things each time you practice a routine with a resident. Varying words or procedures from practice episode to practice episode makes it more difficult for residents to learn and establish a routine and new habit. It helps if the words that staff members will be using are written down, along with the steps to take in practicing a routine, so that all staff members across all shifts follow a consistent caring routine.

Thus, behaviors can be learned and unlearned. New behaviors can replace old behaviors. Everything depends on awareness that this is possible, and then knowing how to teach persons with dementia effectively. We also must remember that we are dealing with persons, not robots, and that persons with dementia have values, habits, and beliefs that were developed over decades of life experience. As any rehabilitation professional will tell you, it is one thing to provide training and a healthy regimen to a person (with or without dementia) in therapy sessions, and quite another thing for that person to use the training and follow the regimen after the therapy sessions.

Another important thing to remember is this: If persons with dementia can learn new behaviors (and methods of resolving conflict or experiencing empathy for others involve behaviors), persons with dementia should be able to learn some of the same techniques and behaviors that staff can learn. For example, we have trained persons with dementia to lead activities for other persons with dementia. It starts with training a staff member how to lead the activity, then having a resident with dementia become the "assistant" of the staff member. Over time, the resident takes over more and more of the leadership components of the activity, and learns to feel more confident in the role, until the resident can lead the activity with little or no help from staff members (Skrajner *et al.* 2014). In a similar way, modeling conflict resolution and peaceful behaviors for residents, then letting residents have (guided) practice with them, can enable such behaviors to become learned as new habits.

In addition, it is important to view persons with dementia as having a disability rather than a disease (Mast *et al.* 2015). When we take this perspective, we can begin to consider ways to allow persons with dementia to circumvent their disabilities. For example, a woman with dementia who had hearing difficulties was trying to take part in an exercise class. When the staff member leading exercises said, "Touch your toes," the woman could not hear clearly and yelled out, "I don't want to pick my nose!" Other residents began to yell at her, and she started yelling back. One of the authors then pointed to the exercise leader and showed the woman a written message: "Watch her. Do what she does." The woman quieted down, watched the staff member, and began to touch her toes. Everyone calmed down and began doing the exercises together.

The point to this story is that we must use a two-step process to help overcome physical and cognitive deficits in persons with dementia. First, we must understand the reason why a person with dementia is finding a situation challenging. The woman described above was having difficulty hearing, which led to frustration and ultimately to conflict with other residents. The second step is to determine what remaining abilities can be used to circumvent deficits. In this case, her vision and cognitive capacities allowed her to read and understand the words on the card. Using this approach, rather than expecting her to use her impaired hearing, allowed the woman to overcome her deficits, and the conflict with other residents was eliminated.

Again, this is about knowing the persons with dementia—their capacities and their limitations. Frustration and negative behaviors between residents and staff or among residents themselves can be prevented in advance by knowing residents as persons, and thus understanding *why* they react in the ways that they do. A good resource for learning to think like a detective to understand why persons with dementia do what they do, and to match the cause of a behavior with an intervention, is found in the book *Hiding the Stranger in the Mirror* (Camp 2012), which is listed in the Bibliography.[1]

---

1   It can be acquired on our website (www.cen4ard.com).

CHAPTER 4

TEACHING EMPATHY

Empathy has been studied in adults of different ages, and is broken down into two components: cognitive empathy and affective empathy. Cognitive empathy refers to a conscious understanding of how another person is feeling by looking at their facial expressions, body language, etc., and making an inference based on those cues. Affective empathy involves an unconscious understanding of another's feelings, shown when a person resonates with and shares the same feeling that the person is seeing in another person (Hühnel *et al.* 2014). It is possible to not have cognitive/conscious empathy for someone else's emotion, but still have an unconscious understanding and empathy for that emotion in another.

For example, Hühnel and colleagues (2014) found that older adults were not as accurate as younger adults in consciously "decoding" videos of happy or sad facial expressions, but were equally likely to unconsciously mimic the facial expressions of happiness or sadness. Since unconscious mental processing is often preserved in persons with dementia, as we discussed in Chapter 3, it would make sense that persons with dementia also could exhibit empathy, at least unconsciously.

This is related to a finding that persons with advanced dementia, who may not consciously recognize their own reflection in a mirror, may still recognize themselves unconsciously. For example, while in front of a mirror, they may have a conversation with their reflection, indicating a lack of conscious self-recognition. But at the same time, they may be combing their hair, indicating an unconscious self-recognition and using their reflection to help groom themselves (Bologna and Camp 1997). In addition, these persons were able to temporarily regain conscious self-recognition through interventions (such as labeling the mirror as "Mirror").

There are two important implications of these findings. The first is that persons with dementia may, indeed, be able to feel and exhibit empathy for others' feelings. The second is that, since persons with dementia can learn, it may be possible to build on their empathetic abilities and expand their capacity to experience empathy for others' feelings. How might this be done?

Let us examine two situations where empathy training would be useful. In the first, a person with early stage dementia makes insulting or disparaging remarks about a person with more advanced dementia, even to the face of the more impaired individual. The key to this situation is to understand why this is happening. Often, this type of behavior is seen because of fear. The person who is less impaired is afraid of becoming like the person who is more impaired. One typical way of dealing with such fear is to "distance" oneself from the situation. This is done by creating a "me" versus "them" division—"I am not like him/her/them and I never will be. They are different than me—sicker/less intelligent/less capable—and I will *never* be like them." This is a coping mechanism, but it does much harm. In addition, as the more capable person advances in dementia, this way of thinking can lead to self-loathing and despair.

The first thing to do is to talk with the person who is insulting or denigrating the other resident. Ask the person how they would feel if someone said such things to them. Ask them how the person receiving the insults must feel when hearing such things. If the higher functioning person has religious or spiritual beliefs based on treating others the way you wish to be treated, these ideas can be brought into the discussion.

The next step is to find a way for the higher functioning individual to help or assist the lower functioning person. For example, we have seen instances where a woman who had difficulty feeding herself began to be assisted by a resident who previously had made hurtful comments about the woman's impairments. It is important for residents to see each other as persons, and to foster relationships among themselves, especially when they are at different stages of dementia and/or physical capabilities. When a more impaired resident thanks another resident for assistance provided, or for their company, it humanizes the situation and enables residents to see other residents as persons.

Another scenario involves a group of residents who refuse to accept a new resident into their group or community. They may say to a new resident, "Go away. This seat is taken," or, "You are not wanted here," or, if there is some racial or cultural difference between members of the group and the newcomer, "Your kind are not welcome here. Go back to where you came from."

In this situation, as always, it helps to think about why this is happening. Excluding people who are "different" is a common social behavior. It feeds on itself, until it becomes a habit. Such habits can be hard to break, especially when persons have dementia. Again, the first thing to do is to talk with the persons who are excluding the new resident and ask how they would feel if this happened to them. As before, it can be useful to invoke religious or spiritual beliefs involving treating others as we want to be treated.

While this may initially get the group to agree to change or to treat the new resident better, there remain the challenges of changing habits in light of memory loss associated with dementia. The members of the group may forget the conversation about fair treatment and revert to old habits. This is where new, unconscious learning can be used. For example, we have described a situation where a group of white women in a memory care program were hurtful to a new male client who was African American. When it was pointed out that such behavior was not "Christian," they agreed and said they would change. However, they quickly forgot the conversation and their behaviors toward the man did not change. Staff then gave the man the role of handing out prizes for games and contests, so that he was giving prizes to women of this group on a regular basis. This created a classical conditioning situation, in which the positive emotions experienced by winning a prize were repeatedly associated with this gentleman. In this way, members of the group learned to like this man in an automatic, unconscious process.

Of course, the best way to create empathy is to create an empathetic social and physical environment. As we discuss in more detail in Chapter 8, this involves creating rules of behavior that are accepted and enforced by group members. In addition, it is important to practice these behaviors on a regular basis. Empathetic behaviors can become new habits, and new habits can be learned by persons with dementia. For example, a welcoming ceremony for new residents can become part of a dementia care community's standard practice. When new people arrive, they can introduce themselves and tell a bit about themselves, and other residents can find areas of common interest with them.

A reading group activity can involve the group reading aloud a story that focuses on events in the life of the new person to get to know the person better (if that is okay with the new resident).

Another useful approach is to have special days for the community to celebrate the cultural diversity of its members, for example, a day celebrating all things Irish, or Mexican, etc. Food, music, dress or costumes, guest speakers, games, explanations and examples of customs, etc., can have a specific cultural theme. Note that this can extend to the cultures of staff members as well. Celebrating diversity and gaining a better understanding of another's way of life is a useful way to promote respect and empathy within a community. It helps to take photos of these celebrations and put them into books or albums that staff members and residents can refer back to, a means of maintaining the effects of this approach.

CHAPTER 5

CONFLICT RESOLUTION

Mahatma Gandhi, who was a friend of Maria Montessori and greeted her when she came to India, said that peace is not the absence of conflict but the ability to cope with it. Conflict arises from many causes: unmet needs (Cohen-Mansfield 2015), misunderstandings, different values/perceptions, jealousy, etc. Note that these are the same causes for conflict among "normal" people; these are human experiences, familiar to everyone. Remember that a person with dementia is a normal person who has disabilities in cognition. And as is true for everyone, all conflict resolution requires communication among all parties.

Enabling persons with dementia to cope with conflict is a three-part process. First, as we discussed in Chapter 1, we must be good role models of peace-loving persons. Second, we must become good mediators of conflicts. Third, we must train persons with dementia to acquire the behaviors necessary to resolve conflict among themselves.

As we mentioned earlier, peace begins within ourselves. Similarly, the ability to manage conflict must begin within ourselves, and a first step is to be able to control our own emotions. One technique for doing this is the SOSS approach. How you use the approach will vary depending on the context, but SOSS refers to Stop—Oxygenate—Safe Place—Strong Solutions. This is a way to regain control over your emotions, and to allow you to focus on finding solutions to challenges that are producing stress for you. The first step—Stop—involves making a conscious effort to stop your train of thought. If you do not stop, you are pulled into a reactionary mode and it is easy for your thoughts and behaviors to escalate into conflict; you "go out of control" with little hope of a positive resolution to your situation.

Often when we are stressed we tend to perseverate in our thinking—to keep rehashing what we think is wrong or distressing—so all our concentration is on our negative feelings and our worry about what might happen, with our thoughts repeating themselves over and over again. Thus, we have to break this thought pattern. We must stop thinking about the problem or whatever is giving us stress and take a "time out" for ourselves.

Next, we must take some deep breaths ("Oxygenate"), focusing our attention on how the air comes into us and then leaves us when we breathe. When we are stressed we go into a "fight or flight" mode, and our breath becomes quick and shallow. Deep breathing oxygenates the brain, and enables the body and brain to relax.

The third step is to take ourselves, in our mind, to a safe place—to a place and time when we felt calm and happy. For example, we might think of a beach or the woods where we walked and felt tranquil and at ease. We might remember and see the image of a time when we were with good friends or were playing with a young child or grandchild. Taking ourselves to a safe place further calms us down and "centers" us—it reminds us of what is important to us in life and helps put current "crises" in perspective. Shortly, we also will discuss creating a physical "safe place" where conflicts can be resolved. In addition, a common mindfulness mantra can be helpful, something like "Let me be safe." It is only when we have a feeling of safety that we are free to explore options fully and to let go of a defensive or attack mode of thinking.

Finally, once we are calm, we can begin to think about solutions or things to try or at least ways of putting our current problems and situations into a different context. Most things that make us stressed really are not "life or death" situations, though we often react as if they were. At this point we can more objectively look at why we were so distressed and decide on next steps without doing so in a panic. We also can learn to see what started the panic, and learn to stop the anxiety cascade before it gets out of control. More information about this approach can be found in Appendix 5.

Of course, the SOSS approach is a set of procedures, and people can be trained so they become a habit. As we discussed in Chapter 3, persons with dementia can be trained to learn new procedures and habits, so this approach also could be used with residents with dementia. Also, the SOSS approach is one of many available to assist in dealing with emotions. In Chapter 6 we discuss Mindfulness, which can be useful for both staff mediators as well as residents with dementia.

BEING A GOOD MEDIATOR

First, it is important to establish "ground rules" for discussions and exchanges during mediation. While persons are allowed to disagree and to express their emotions, this must be done in a respectful way. Learning how to express emotions appropriately, especially negative ones such as anger, may be a challenge for residents. They may respond in different ways, such as not wanting to express any emotions or being all too ready to "dump" their negative feelings on someone else.

An example of respectful expression of emotion is the use of fair fighting techniques. These are methods that enable persons to express disagreements and feelings without attacking or insulting the other person. For example, using "I" messages rather than "You" messages is emphasized. It is important to use "I" statements, such as "I think that..." or "When you did that I felt..." This is different than "You" statements, such as "You are unreasonable" or "You did a bad thing." When a person uses "You" statements, it is a way of assigning blame to the other person.

A person whose idea has been rejected disrespectfully might learn to respond: "When you say 'That's stupid,' I feel hurt and just want to leave." This allows the person who was insulted to express his or her feelings and give feedback without attacking the other person. That is very different than saying, "You started this!" or "You should have kept your mouth shut," or "Oh yeah? Well, you're even more stupid!" "You" messages assign blame and cause defenses to go up. The last example also reflects another rule of fair fighting—no name calling. Name calling does nothing to help resolve conflict, and it usually creates greater barriers to finding a resolution. Resources for rules of fair fighting are shown in Appendix 3. Again, these are procedures that can be practiced in advance so that they are familiar to residents when applied in a mediation session. In addition, it is important to practice feeling empathy, as discussed in Chapter 4. If a person cannot feel empathy towards another, then hearing that a remark hurt another's feelings does not have the desired effect.

Once mediation is started, the mediator must gather information. By attentively listening and not interrupting, the mediator allows everyone to express their thoughts and feelings without judgment while modeling respectful behavior for the residents. This helps draw out the underlying issues of the conflict, which may or may not be involved with the current situation. The mediator also must pay attention to nonverbal communications, which are important sources of information.

Detective work and knowing the residents, along with some skills in diplomacy, are important for successful mediation. People come with different backgrounds, nationalities, social conventions, etc. Because of these differences among individuals, disagreements and conflicts happen. Knowing a person's background, their likes and dislikes and "hot points," helps to understand and diffuse a situation before it leads to conflicts. And when conflicts do arise, it is important to focus on the humanity of the person disagreeing with you. Disagreements are a part of life, but how we handle disagreements determines how we live.

While the mediator must reinforce appropriate and positive responses, it is critical that the mediator not take sides. The mediator must be a neutral party, with the role of assisting the residents to resolve a conflict and develop a better relationship with one another. The mediator should stay out of power struggles—keep redirecting discussion back to resolving a conflict—and remind the residents that both people may need to compromise (maintaining a relationship is most important when resolving conflict). This illustrates the idea of creating a "win–win" outcome.

Individuals in conflict face each other with the mediator between them. It is critical that, as mediator, you focus on creating a "win–win" scenario for the residents in conflict. This emphasizes cooperation among individuals. A "winner" leaves feeling good, a "loser" leaves with self-esteem deflated, as if they had not been heard and their feelings ignored. A win–win requires discussion on both sides, respect, and agreement to solve problems mutually. The process is about finding a solution, not assigning blame, an approach that must be established from the start. It may help to have a "mediation corner" or "mediation room" as the place where these activities take place, with posters and slogans emphasizing the messages of "win–win" and cooperation. (We discuss creating features of physical environments to facilitate conflict resolution in more detail in Chapter 8.) Peacemaking, in ourselves and in others, involves creating a sense of trust and comfort.

BEHAVIORS TO PRACTICE DURING CONFLICT RESOLUTION EPISODES

It also is useful for the mediator to state the problem or conflicting sides of a disagreement in an objective way, so that all parties can agree about the basis of the conflict. Statements made during discussions may need to be written on a flip chart, so that everyone can see (and not have to remember) what has been said. Given that the persons in conflict have dementia, putting this in writing makes it difficult to misinterpret or forget. Also, seeing one's words can be a useful type of feedback, and the speaker may wish to edit or modify harsh or illogical or unreasonable statements when seen in "black and white."

Listening

When a person makes a statement, the mediator may ask the other individual to state what they think they heard, as a way of teaching better listening and understanding. Listening is the highest form of respect. Being listened to is very valuable in and of itself, and is an important part of the process. It acknowledges the worth of the person speaking (with or without dementia). Positive feelings can come from being listened to, but sometimes appropriate listening involves behaviors that must and can be learned, even by older adults, even if they have dementia. So, as a first step, the mediator must model appropriate listening.

One of the keys to good listening is not to interrupt when someone else is speaking. At the start of a discussion, each person is reminded of the rules (which are written down and visually present) and takes turns telling their side of the story, while the other person listens. Being listened to also helps the speaker be understood for who this person is and why they reacted as they did. (Sometimes it may help to give residents practice listening outside of a conflict situation, or to do some role playing that involves listening as part of community-building activities. We discuss role playing in more detail later in this chapter.)

Finding solutions

When both sides have spoken, the mediator says, "How can we resolve this matter? What can you do to move past this?" Once people agree as to what the conflict is about, it is easier to suggest possible solutions if needed. Solutions should be put in writing, which is important for a variety of reasons. When persons are looking at the same printed words, it is more difficult to have misconceptions or different memories of what was agreed upon. This is especially critical for persons with memory impairment. In addition, the agreement should be dated and end with a statement that says "everyone agrees to this" with all parties including the mediator signing the agreement. If a resident does not remember the meeting (or claims not to remember the meeting), and the solution that mutually was agreed to, having a signature in their handwriting on the document is the best evidence that these are the terms that all persons agreed to honor. This is especially helpful if a conflict and its causes are repeated. At that point, it may become necessary to change the physical or social environments as a means of preventing future conflicts.

Never try to argue with a person who has memory impairment by saying a thing happened which they cannot remember. Logic is on their side. This is true for any person—if you cannot remember that something happened then in your mind it did not happen. There must be other evidence (including, perhaps, a photo of everyone signing the agreement and shaking hands) that an event occurred beyond a verbal agreement.

Finally, it requires creativity to find solutions that satisfy both persons' needs—something that is realistic and doable. The goal of the mediator should be to encourage and enable the residents to come up with their own solution that is mutually agreed upon. This is much better than trying to impose a solution; and when residents create a solution, they are more capable of doing so again if other disagreements arise. This is about empowering both parties, and creating habits and attitudes that may eventually enable conflicts to be resolved without a mediator, or even to prevent a conflict from occurring in the first place. The mediator who is not needed has done the best job, for that mediator has worked with residents to enable them to resolve conflicts on their own.

Cool off periods

Sometimes a situation may arise where anger and other emotions are so powerful or the situation is so complicated that an agreement cannot be reached in that moment. In these cases, persons in disagreement can agree to disagree. Where anger is intense, it helps to separate the persons involved. "Cool down" locations or "Tranquility Rooms" can be used to let people's emotions calm down. It may help to say, "Let's stop for today. We can think more about this overnight, and what we can try to do to make things better, and then meet again here tomorrow. Is that okay for you? Can we agree to come back tomorrow and try again?"

Apologizing and forgiveness

To have long-lasting effects, and create a peaceful community, the conflict resolution process must also involve apologizing and forgiveness. These allow persons to "get past" a conflict and reduce the likelihood of holding grudges. Even in persons with memory deficits, getting to a solution that includes apologizing and forgiveness ends the process with all parties feeling better about themselves and each other.

These behaviors may feel odd or uncomfortable to some people, especially if they had positions of authority in their homes or places of business. As always, it helps to model and practice these behaviors outside of the conflict situation beforehand. Apologizing is a way of saying that a person is sorry for the thing they did or said, and for the hurt it may have caused. "I am sorry that the thing I said offended you" is a typical example, as is "I apologize that what I did hurt you." Apologizing is a first step, and a good place to start. An apology acknowledges that what you did or said might have caused pain or harm.

A second and more challenging step is to ask the other person for forgiveness. This gives control to the other person, who may or may not say that they forgive you. When you apologize, you are simply stating something. When you ask for forgiveness, you are requesting absolution. Learning to ask for and to give forgiveness can be difficult for anyone, but it also can bring about healing and be life-affirming. This step in the process, again, should be practiced ahead of time and discussed outside of the heat of argument or disagreement during a conflict situation. Once more, it helps if the mediator also models and practices this for the residents.

Role playing

Behaviors associated with peace and conflict resolution, like all behaviors, can be learned. They may seem strange at first to some residents (or staff members), but practicing them, like practicing any behaviors, makes such behaviors become "normal" and routine. While having an intellectual understanding of the underlying concepts involved is helpful, this is not necessary. If persons behave in peaceful and cooperative ways, their understanding of the underlying concepts of peace and cooperation is not critical to their ability to display these behaviors. Likewise, persons who understand the concepts of peace and cooperation may behave in ways that are contradictory to these ideas. Such contradictory behavior may be a conscious rejection of these ideas ("Others cooperate, we compete" "Give war a chance"), an attempt to justify the contradiction ("This is just doing business"), or something done unconsciously ("Was that really bullying?"). The point is that persons with (and without) dementia can learn peacefulness. However, like any behaviors, the learning will involve appropriate training and practice.

Role playing is a very effective and often necessary training method for teaching peacefulness and conflict resolution. The best way to learn a behavior is to do it, not just think about it. Role playing gives persons practice while creating the context in which the behavior should take place. For example, during a committee meeting of residents with dementia, time can be set aside to practice how committee members should act if there is a disagreement among members. A hypothetical scenario can be presented, the rules for dealing with disagreements made visibly available, and the appropriate way to respectfully disagree can be practiced. Again, it takes time to practice alternatives to conflict, so this requires a commitment of time on the part of staff and residents. However, to do nothing is worse and can be much more damaging to the social environment and relationships among members of a community. Unresolved conflicts allow anger, resentments, and disrespect towards others to linger and grow over time.

Spaced-retrieval

As we mentioned in Chapter 3, practice enables persons with dementia to learn new habits and associations. One especially efficient form of practice, for role playing or any other learning goal, is called spaced-retrieval (Camp 2006b). Spaced-retrieval involves giving someone practice successfully remembering information over longer and longer periods of time. For example, if you wished to help a group of residents learn the SOSS technique, you might practice in this way. First, you would discuss the approach with them and ask if they thought it would be a good idea to try to learn it. If they agreed, you would start by saying that it helps to break things down into steps. Then you could have them practice the Stop and Oxygenate components of the technique. You might say, "What do we do first if we are anxious or upset?" Then you would tell them, "Stop and Oxygenate." Next, you would say again, "Now, what do we do first if we are anxious or upset?" The group would then answer, "Stop and Oxygenate." This represents immediate recall, which is usually available to persons with dementia. They have a window in which new information still is available in short-term memory. Then you have them practice the Stop and Oxygenate procedure (breathing, etc.).

Next, you would wait for about 30 seconds, filling this interval with small talk, and repeat the question, having the group give their response and practice the procedure as in the example above. Intervals would be expanded with each practice, using a schedule such as immediate recall, 30 second interval, 60 second interval, two minute interval, four minute interval, eight minute interval, etc. The time intervals between asking about Stop and Oxygenate would be spent doing other things, such as activities or discussion about other topics. If residents have difficulty remembering the answer, for example, after eight minutes have elapsed since the last question about the procedure, then you provide them with the correct answer and next ask the question immediately afterwards (giving a chance at immediate recall). This lets every recall trial end in a correct response. The next interval is shortened to the one that produced a correct response, such as four minutes in this case. The length of the following interval can be tried again at eight minutes. If this proves difficult, intervals can be expanded at a slower rate (e.g. four minutes, six minutes, eight minutes). The key is to ensure that recalls are successful. It is our experience that once persons with memory difficulties can retain information for over 10–12 minutes, the information begins to move into long-term memory.

Practice with the first steps of SOSS can continue, with the question being asked at the start of each session. When the group seems to be answering well at the start of a few sessions, the next step of the SOSS process can be added to the training, and when it is mastered, the last step added using the same approach. Of course, spaced-retrieval can be used to train individuals with dementia as well as groups for a variety of procedures and associations (Bourgeois *et al.* 2003;

Camp 2006b; Camp, Bird and Cherry 2000). Additional information and resources concerning spaced-retrieval are provided in Appendix 5, and on our website.[1]

The talking stick

One way to teach listening without interruption is with the use of an object, such as a talking stick. The object can be anything (ideally an object chosen by residents). In the case of a talking stick, a resident who wishes to speak raises their hand and is given the talking stick to hold. Whoever is holding the talking stick gets to speak, while the others in the group listen. Then the stick is handed to the next speaker. One advantage of creating this procedure is that the external aid of the talking stick and the repetition of the behavior (only the person holding the stick can talk, while everyone else listens) makes it an ideal way for persons with dementia to learn not only how to use the talking stick, but also how to listen without interruption.

A second advantage of this procedure is that when it is practiced in group settings, such as a committee meeting of residents who decided where the community would like to go for outings, the talking stick already is familiar when used during a conflict resolution meeting with a mediator. Thus, the habit of listening when someone else holds the talking stick can be carried over to this peace-making process, facilitating discussion and work toward a solution.

WHEN A PEACE METHOD IS CHALLENGED

Challenges to conflict resolution often come from past behavior or cultural beliefs, stereotypes, assumptions, and

---

1   www.cen4ard.com

habitual ways of thinking. Some persons see peacefulness, asking forgiveness, compromise, or cooperation as signs of weakness. Others, who perhaps have challenges experiencing empathy, may genuinely believe that they have not insulted or injured another person, or that the other person misinterpreted what was said or done to them. Common rejections of the peace method are expressed along the lines of:

- they are too sensitive

- they need to toughen up

- I did not do that—they are lying

- I did not say that—they are lying

- if they can't take the heat, get out of the kitchen

- this is who I am, take it or leave it.

Community guidelines

To address challenges to peace methods, it is important to have a list of guidelines for a community or family or household. Throughout our lives we live with rules that society provides to enable us to live "civilly"—in a community. Stop signs, traffic signals, "walk/don't walk" signs, "no parking here" signs, and other laws are designed to enable a diverse set of individuals to be able to live together more safely. Obeying rules (written and unwritten) is a natural and accepted habit of persons with dementia, and rules also provide ways of civilly resolving conflicts when they arise.

These guidelines should be discussed by all stakeholders, agreed to and signed off on in advance. For residential settings such as assisted living or skilled nursing, these community rules should be shown to family members of new residents and to new residents themselves, and agreed to, before someone moves into the community. This process achieves several important things:

- it emphasizes that "equality" and "fairness" are key values that will be guiding future interactions for everyone, and that everyone will be held to the same standards for showing respect and cooperation

- it creates the expectation that everyone will be trusted and will keep their promises

- it emphasizes that the environment should allow everyone to feel safe

- it demonstrates that everyone will be treated the same

- it describes consequences for behaviors that are not appropriate

- it emphasizes that consequences are the result of choices made by residents, and that good choices are expected to be the norm for the community.

Guidelines should explain methods of dealing with conflict in a routine manner. We offer some examples of guidelines in Appendix 2. It helps, before any gathering in which there will be discussions and potential disagreements or differences of opinion, to first go over the guidelines. As always, these rules should be displayed for everyone to see. This provides an exercise in how to discuss important topics and come to a mutually accepted agreement.

DEALING WITH PHYSICAL AGGRESSION
When a physically aggressive act has occurred, such as a resident hitting another resident, there needs to be a set procedure in place to deal with the situation immediately.

First, the residents must be separated. Safety is the primary issue, and residents must be kept out of harm's way. Next, the person who committed the physically aggressive act should be given an evaluation. This should involve assessment of pain, infection, and any other physical issue, in combination with dementia, that could precipitate an aggressive act. Additionally, it needs to be determined whether the offending resident has any psychiatric issues, and if so, how they should be treated. There should also be a discussion with the resident to determine if the resident is aware of what happened or not, can describe their motivation for the physical aggression or not, etc. Staff must investigate and determine what exactly triggered the aggressive act—this is critical for developing action plans to prevent the recurrence of this behavior.

This situation is comparable in many ways to dealing with physical aggression in a school, where entering students are made aware of the rules and consequences for breaking them. Similarly, in residential care, there need to be set rules and consequences for physical violence, which are described and agreed to at the time of admission by family members and, ideally, also by the resident. In addition, as we've said before, it's important to understand the personal history and recent behavior patterns of the resident. This can help with determining the reason for the physical aggression. Further, the effects of the aggression must be considered. Did the aggression result in injury, and if so, what was the extent of injury?

Finally, there should be zero tolerance for a staff member committing an act of physical violence directed toward a resident in memory care.

ACCEPTING THE CHALLENGING RESIDENT

There is a final thing to remember. We must learn to accept challenging persons, and to try to enable them to be integrated into the community as well. This often will be difficult. It is easy to like and work with "nice" individuals who are polite and respectful and happy much of the time. How we respond to challenging persons is a true measure of our commitment to a peaceful, empathetic lifestyle. These are the persons who are easy to reject. In many instances, most of their contact with other persons has involved their being disagreeable.

While it is necessary to put limits on some behaviors such as physical violence, verbal abuse, bullying, etc., we must always try to understand why a person is behaving in such a destructive way. We must work to see the humanity behind their behavior, and do the best we can to try to "bring them around" to a more fulfilling life. Our first instinct when encountering an "unlikeable" person is to avoid them, but we must remember what we tell others about empathy and understanding, applying those principles in this instance as well. As always, we must model for our residents. We must look for the key or the window into the humanity within the person who challenges us and our beliefs.

WORKING WITH PERSONS IN ADVANCED STAGES OF DEMENTIA

Most of the examples and exercises we have presented are relevant for persons with early to moderate stages of dementia. What can we do for persons with more advanced dementia, especially if they have challenges communicating, understanding what is said to them, etc.? Many times, conflicts arise between persons at different stages of dementia. Persons in earlier stages may get angry or impatient when interacting with a person who has more difficulty processing information. Under these circumstances, focusing on the person who is more cognitively intact is helpful. The use of techniques described in Chapter 4 on building empathy can be used with the person in an earlier stage of dementia.

For example, a man in memory care who was very intelligent and in early stage dementia would make fun of a woman in that residence who would perpetually speak about certain animals, and use a particular word in each sentence she spoke. Instead of asking him to stop (he had said that he would on several occasions, and then forgotten the promise), he was asked, "Why do you think she does that?" His initial response was, "Because she's crazy." Then he was told, "You're an intelligent man. Let's think about why a person would do this." A discussion followed about different conditions that might affect how a person speaks, along with the idea that the behavior might not be under conscious control. At the end of the discussion he agreed that, under the circumstances, making fun of a person in such a condition was simply inappropriate and inconsiderate. Interestingly, though he made no promises at the end of the discussion, he stopped his taunting of the woman. We believe that this resulted from creating a sense of empathy for the woman. Simply telling him to stop did not make the same impression. Feelings are more likely to be retained in persons with dementia than words alone.

A memory care resident who was upset and impatient with a woman with more advanced dementia would call her names and say that the woman was "acting crazy." When such behaviors occur, as we have mentioned before, it is important to ask, "Why is this happening?" The answer can never be, "Because they have dementia." This is circular reasoning— "Why is this happening?—Because they have dementia.

How do we know they have dementia?—Because this is happening." Instead, it is most useful to view these as "responsive" behaviors—behaviors that are in response to an unmet human need (Cohen-Mansfield 2015). Again, we refer you to the book *Hiding the Stranger in the Mirror* (Camp 2012) for more information on this topic.

In the case of persons with earlier-stage dementia disparaging persons with more advanced dementia, a common reason for this behavior is fear. These individuals fear that their condition will progress to the point that they will resemble the persons they are disparaging. In addition, these early-stage residents may have accepted the stigma and negative images associated with advanced dementia that are so prevalent in our culture. Thus, as a defense mechanism against these thoughts, these residents at early stages of dementia begin to separate themselves cognitively and emotionally from those with advanced dementia, who are regarded as different, inferior, sick, etc. The humanity of persons being ridiculed is lost, and it becomes easy to treat others as objects rather than human beings. Once this bridge is crossed, indignities can be heaped upon others without pangs of conscience.

We were having dinner in France with a group from a nursing home association, and a physician in the group asked us this question: "Is it possible for a person with advanced dementia to be happy?" A researcher focusing on pharmacologic treatments for dementia recently made the statement that it was sad to think that ultimately persons with dementia lost their humanity. It is little wonder that residents (and sometimes staff members, and even family members) may treat those in more advanced stages of dementia as less than human. This is why the values underlying the Montessori Pledge are so important. We must treat others as we wish to be treated, and enable persons with dementia to do this with each other. We must work to humanize dementia care, overcoming and replacing what Thomas Kitwood (1997) referred to as "toxic social systems."

Another approach is to try to enlist the person in earlier stages of dementia as an assistant or "volunteer" in working with the person with more advanced dementia. For example, a memory care resident was upset and impatient with another woman on the unit who was more advanced in her dementia, and who had difficulty feeding herself. However, when the first resident was asked to become a "volunteer" and to assist in helping the woman eat, and was provided with training in the proper technique, everything changed. Being given a "Volunteer" badge enabled the first resident to get past the self-imposed barrier of staying away from "people like that," because the badge provided evidence that the first resident was like staff members rather than like the woman needing assistance. The first resident began to view the woman as her responsibility, and appreciated both the opportunity to serve another person, as well as the thanks and gratitude she received from the woman being assisted.

In other cases, two memory care residents, one of whom was blind, would argue with each other. However, when the first resident began to spend time reading to the blind resident, it changed the nature of their relationship, and they became friends. A man in memory care who refused to take part in activities with "those people" was asked if he would like to create a short story reading club for the group, and he did so. Each evening he would select props, music, and other items to enliven the discussion of the short story to be read the next day. "Those people" became "my people." These are examples of enabling persons with early stage dementia to see the humanity in residents with more advanced dementia.

Classical conditioning

As we discussed when talking about a "preemptive nice," it is possible for persons with dementia to learn unconsciously through a process of classical conditioning. For example, if a resident with advanced dementia has pain due to arthritis, a hip replacement, etc., and a staff member tries to get the resident out of bed, the resident can begin to associate this staff member with the increase in pain caused by the movement. The staff member can be viewed as a persecutor and tormentor. This also can occur during provision of personal care such as bringing a resident into the bathroom or providing a shower.

Fortunately, positive associations can be learned as well. First, it always helps for staff members to introduce themselves, and to let the resident know why they are there and what is going to happen. Talking to the resident with advanced dementia in a calm manner, making eye contact, speaking face-to-face (not talking behind the person with dementia), moving slowly, and demonstrating what is going to happen before doing it, all help keep a situation calm and less likely to result in confrontation.

As in Lamaze training for childbirth, it helps to have residents focus on something outside of themselves during a transfer that might be painful, ideally something positive (such as holding and eating a favorite food, singing along with a favorite song, etc.). This creates positive associations with the staff member. Alternatively, there may be a way to deliver care without moving the resident, as in providing an in-bed "massage" with rinseless soap. Resources such as "Bathing without a Battle" and "Mouth Care without a Battle" are extremely helpful in this regard, and are listed in Appendix 5.

In another case, a man with advanced dementia was aggressive throughout the day and in a variety of different environments. When this happens, often the cause is internal, and again pain is a typical cause. It was found that he had dental problems resulting in pain. (A clue was that he would hold his jaw with one hand while striking out with the other hand.) To reduce conflict in this situation, the intervention involved treating his dental issues.

External environmental triggers

Another key element in working with persons with advanced dementia is to determine if there are environmental triggers likely to set off aggressive or confrontational behaviors. This also is discussed in detail elsewhere (Camp 2012). For example, a woman with advanced dementia in a memory residence had been living relatively peacefully there for a few years. Then, a man with early-stage dementia came to live there. When he was eating his first lunch in the community, the woman came up behind him and smacked him on the head with a long-handled ladle. She proceeded to follow him throughout the day, trying to hit him. When staff members asked her why she wanted to hurt the man, she said, "He's a guard. Don't you recognize him?"

The woman had been in a concentration camp in World War II, and this man's face reminded her of a guard at the camp. Trying to "reason" with her and convince her that he was not a guard had no effect (and, of course, she would forget these conversations). The key, then, was to find a way to change the trigger. It was learned that the man had been a sailor, and so staff members asked him if he would mind wearing a sailor hat when he was outside of his room. This was put into his plan of care. When he wore the hat, his appearance changed for the woman resident so she believed he was with the navy and was "safe."

Residents with advanced dementia also may have difficulty handling highly stimulating environments. Noisy, crowded, "busy" environments can cause these persons to become agitated and go into a "fight or flight" mode. As a result, they can become aggressive and combative towards persons around them. In this case, the key is to determine which settings are likely to produce these responses and then provide alternatives (such as letting such residents view activities at a distance or providing optional calmer programming).

A man residing in a memory care residence became angry with some of his neighbors, and began to threaten them with physical violence. He came from a background that included serving in the military and was a very strict Roman Catholic. Knowing this, staff asked him if it was appropriate for a man to hit a girl. He answered, "Of course not. That would be wrong and cowardly." The man then was informed that the residents he was threatening were girls (since they were female). Thus, since the behavior of threating women with physical violence was counter to his self-image, he stopped his threats. Whenever his old behavior began to manifest itself, staff would just say, "They're girls," and this would stop his threats again.

In a similar way, we often see older women in memory care get angry and begin to curse staff or other residents with words, as is sometimes said, that would make a sailor blush. What is surprising is that these same women often view themselves as "ladies" who never would use such language, and when informed of what they had said reply, "I would *never* say such a thing!" Why would this happen? Let us examine this pattern of behavior, knowing what we do about dementia.

First, it often is the case that when persons are angry the words spoken are spontaneous and may be said without conscious attention or thinking about what will be said in advance of speaking. Cursing, thus, can be a reflexive and somewhat unconscious form of emotional expression. This is seen especially in persons who have had a stroke and lost the ability to speak sentences, but who still utter curse words when angry. Second, in the case of persons with dementia, the reflexive nature of cursing combined with both a short-term memory loss and the discrepancy between cursing and one's self-image can lead to the ladies' behavior described above.

An intervention to try in the heat of the moment is to say to women such as those we have described when they are cursing, "Please tell me what you are saying." This does two things: 1) it stops the cursing, because they now must process what was said to them and respond; 2) when conscious attention is paid to the utterances, they will stop cursing (as long as such words are considered at odds with their self-image). An alternative approach is to ask them to write down what they want to say. Once again, this forces conscious attention to be paid to their words while also stopping their cursing while they contemplate what to do.

These examples illustrate the need to know the person. Again, behaviors such as saying, "They're girls" or, "Please tell me what you are saying" can be taught to residents as well, so that they also can help in short-circuiting aggressive behaviors in their neighbors. Of course, the best approach in the long run is to examine the situations that are involved in these aggressive actions and to create alternatives that will keep these incidents from arising in the first place.

Keeping apart

As a last resort, there are times when people just do not seem to like one another due to differences in personality, ways of looking at the world, etc. This has little or nothing to do with dementia, and can be seen among family members, co-workers, and anywhere else in the world. Often in our lives we have had to work with persons whom we did not agree with or admire. That is the nature of living in social systems. But we can and do learn to at least tolerate one another, and work or live together in spite of these differences. It is the same for persons with dementia. Sometimes the best way to prevent conflicts among residents is to keep persons separated so they do not "get on each other's nerves."

Imagine a dinner party or wedding reception that you must help plan. A wide variety of individuals will be attending, some of whom like one another, and some who do not. You try to arrange the seating so that you will have an agreeable event, with few instances of friction or argument among your guests. You hope that persons sitting near one another will converse, enjoy each other's company, and have a good experience. The same approach can be taken when residents with dementia will be attending an activity, eating a meal, etc. It helps to know the individuals and their dynamics in such settings. For meals, name tents can be used to arrange seating. Small groups of like-minded people can work together in activities. While we wish that "everyone would get along and like one another," persons with dementia are very human and because they retain their humanity, we must accommodate their foibles just as we would do for any group of persons entering our own homes. Therefore, as we continually work with residents to cultivate a more peaceful and empathetic life, we also must deal with people as they are today.

CHAPTER 6

MINDFULNESS FOR PERSONS WITH DEMENTIA

A discussion of mindfulness (Langer 2014) could take up an entire book (or two) by itself, but we want to provide an introduction to this idea here as it relates to conflict resolution. Mindfulness has rapidly become a popular practice in Western culture, as depicted on the June 2014 cover of *Time* magazine entitled "Mindful Revolution." Derived from Buddhist practices involving meditation, mindfulness involves focusing attention and being in the present moment. It involves a high level of self-awareness—you can step back and observe yourself, your feelings, your thoughts—that is nonjudgmental. Mindfulness creates positive attitudes such as trust, curiosity, generosity, and patience. It allows one to see the world and those around us in an open and accepting way. Practicing mindfulness leads to a welcoming of new experiences and new information.

It should be expected that in a community of persons who practice mindfulness, bitter disputes and conflicts are less likely to occur. As always, this is true for persons with and without dementia. And, once again, we must think about how to allow persons with the cognitive impairments associated with dementia to be able to acquire and enjoy the benefits of mindfulness.

Sometimes persons with dementia are described as "living in the moment," since it is assumed that they do not remember the past well and have difficulty looking into the future. Although those assumptions often are not true, especially on an individual basis, the extent to which time frames become more constricted for persons with dementia could serve as an advantage for them in acquiring mindfulness. Also, it sometimes is assumed that persons with dementia cannot focus and sustain their attention. The same argument is made of young children. And yet, we have seen three-year-old children sustain their attention for extended time frames and be totally oblivious to what is happening around them when they are working in a Montessori classroom. Maria Montessori focused on concentration and its ability to lead to a state of "normalization," which involves being a contributing member of society (Lillard 2011).

We have seen the same thing in older adults with dementia when engaging in meaningful activity within a variety of dementia care settings. Older adults with dementia have successfully engaged in activities such as dance, singing, writing, discussions, volunteering, and spending time with children, as well as in "exotic" activities such as beer making and Tai Chi. Our experience shows that, with a bit of imagination and knowledge on the part of the caregiver, older adults with dementia can participate in, and benefit from, mindfulness exercises.

Here are some of the benefits for persons with dementia who take part in mindfulness programs: reducing stress/ anxiety (meditation of any kind generally produces this effect for almost everyone); helping to regulate emotions; coping better with dementia (especially through learning to let things go); helping with pain control (it's not about getting rid of pain, but learning to cope with it more effectively); and improving interpersonal relations. Mindfulness is used to treat addictions and reduce cravings and other unhealthy behaviors. Learning to appreciate the moment, see the good in others and in oneself, becoming more comfortable with yourself and others, becoming less judgmental—all of these things lead to a better quality of life and the ability to live more peacefully.

Examples of mindfulness exercises include meditations (both while relaxed and while moving, such as when walking), having a "beginner's mind" (learning how to experience something familiar as if experiencing it for the first time), focusing attention, and letting residents see that their experiences are "normal" and a shared part of all human existence. Resources that provide more detailed information about mindfulness exercises and training activities are listed in Appendix 4.

As we mentioned in Chapter 3, it is possible for persons with dementia to learn to lead activities for groups of persons with dementia. The same is true of mindfulness exercises. In its simplest form, a recorded session for guided meditation could be set up and started by a resident. Scripted exercises could be led by residents as well. Of course, with practice, persons with dementia can learn routines such as focusing attention on different parts of the body, exercises such as walking meditation, etc. Once again, when persons with dementia are given control over an activity and make it their own, the activity is more likely to take place and become a routine than if the activity's scheduling and execution is the responsibility of staff or volunteers.

CHAPTER 7

BUILDING THE PEACEFUL ENVIRONMENT

To have peaceful residents, it is necessary to create environments that support peace. This involves both the physical and social environments working in coordination with each other. Especially in the case of persons with dementia, residents must feel safe and in control of their lives. In addition, they must have a sense of belonging to a community, where they know their neighbors and make contributions to the life of their community.

Once again, it is important to make a distinction between an environment that is totally free of conflict because there is no living going on there, and an environment that has living, contributing individuals who may sometimes disagree or come into conflict. The first environment is not "peaceful" in the true sense (as per the U.N. statement on peace in Chapter 2).

We once had a visitor from another country come to our home city. He was the owner of a business involved in long-term care. We had him tour a residence for memory care where the environment was very tranquil, and he remarked that this was a different experience for him, because he heard no screaming. Then we took him to a residence that has been our pilot and prototype for resident-driven communities in memory care—Helen's Place.

This was October, and the residents had decided to go on an outing to pick apples which they would then turn into apple sauce to be served at dinner that evening. When we arrived with our guest, the scene was relatively chaotic. People were talking to each other across the room, asking who they would be driving with, who else was going in which automobile, where was the family member driving each group, etc. The place was far from tranquil, but our visitor remarked, "I see the difference. Here they are living."

We once consulted with Alzheimer's Australia Victoria on a project to train staff members of adult day centers (called "programmed activity groups" there) for persons with dementia in the application of Montessori methods. The project was independently evaluated by researchers from LaTrobe University, who made observations before staff training at the centers and several times afterwards. The researchers' first observation after training was striking—the clients with dementia were much noisier. This was because clients now had assumed responsibility for preparing and serving morning tea for themselves. Clients were talking to one another, assigning jobs, asking about preferences for food and drink, etc. Previously, staff members had served clients, who generally sat and did not speak to one another.

This is not to say that chaos is the norm in a peaceful community, but conversation and activity do reflect the behaviors of persons who know each other, communicate regularly, and coordinate their activities. Their activities are perceived as important and having value, by others and by themselves. Consider a meal eaten in silence versus one with conversation. Which one makes you feel more at ease (at least if the conversation is civil and interesting)?

In a resident-driven community, as we mentioned in an earlier example, there is a welcoming ceremony for new residents, an exemplary exercise in empathy. Imagine waking up in a new place, and realizing you cannot remember where you are or how you got there. (Those of us who travel frequently, especially to other continents, can relate to this feeling very easily.) Someone knocks on your door and says, "Hello. I'm here to help you get dressed and give you a shower." Once you work through that situation, you must find a place to eat. You notice that you don't have any money or credit cards. You now are expected to sit down among a group of strangers, accept food (which you did not select) and wonder when you will be asked to pay for a meal that you think you do not have the means to pay for. This happens every day around the world when a new resident moves into a memory care residence. Many times, the result is isolation, feelings of anger or of being abandoned, and an unwillingness to leave one's own room. Aggressive behavior may follow, directed towards staff or other residents, which in turn often is treated pharmacologically.

Now imagine that when you arrive, you are greeted by a welcoming committee of residents. They bring you a welcome basket (which they created; they also chose the contents of the basket specifically for you). You are read a welcoming speech, and told that this is an "all-inclusive" place where you do not have to pay for food and lodging (it already has been paid for by your family). One of the committee members says, "I will be your friendly neighbor. That means that I will come to get you tomorrow to take you to breakfast and introduce you to people. Don't worry. We are all friendly people here." The next morning, the friendly neighbor knocks on the door, re-introduces himself or herself, and invites you to come to breakfast. You are seated at a chair at the table with a placemat in front of you that says "Welcome home..." and your name comes after "home." Residents, singly or in pairs, come up to you to introduce themselves and to welcome you. After you become acclimated, you are invited to join the welcoming committee to help introduce newer members to the community. This happens every day around the world when a new resident moves into a memory care residence that has embraced the concept of resident-driven communities. Which of these two scenarios would you rather experience?

To be at peace, therefore, the resident must feel safe as well as affirmed for who they are. When we talk to residents in dementia care, we often ask, "What do you want?" Many times, the answer is, "I want people living here to know me, and I want to know them. I want the people working here to know me, and I want to know them." This is a request for community—a place where a person feels that they are known and where they belong. They know their neighbors and are known by them. It is a place where residents care about each other. When a resident comes back from a stay in the hospital, other residents come to their room to welcome them back and to see how they are doing. In the best resident-driven memory care communities, a resident in the hospital is visited by other residents while in the hospital. It is simple, really. A person with dementia wants to live in a way and in a place that persons without dementia would want to live.

As we have mentioned before, the community of residents with dementia should be allowed to create a set of rules for living in the community. It sometimes is assumed that because persons with dementia have this diagnosis, they have become incapable of thinking or reasoning. This is not the case, but it can be made to appear that way when their environment neither offers nor encourages the capacity to have choice, make decisions, or otherwise engage in thinking and reasoning.

THE PHYSICAL ENVIRONMENT

The physical environment for dementia care is an important element in creating peace and empathy. The environment can be constraining and controlling, or inviting and supporting of both independence and respectful social interaction. There are many codes and regulations regarding how to create environments for persons with disabilities, such as the use of ramps for persons with challenges to mobility. Indeed, these are useful when considering how to create supportive environments for persons with dementia. In dementia care, a key environmental element is the ability to give permission to residents to use their environment.

For example, in one memory care residence there was a place to get water. It looked similar to water containers in hotel lobbies, with ice and fruit in a clear container and cups next to it. Generally, staff would be responsible for pouring water from the container and trying to get residents to drink. After training in person-centered care, staff members put up a sign next to the water that said "Help yourself." A resident in a wheelchair immediately said, "It's about time," and went over to get water for herself. Another resident then walked over and said, "Anybody else need some?" and began getting water for other residents. Now the water container must be refilled every afternoon, since residents are drinking more water. There is a "fruit committee" that selects and prepares the fruit to be used in the water the next day. In addition, there has been a significant decrease in urinary tract infections in the memory care residence, because of increased hydration.

This example illustrates several important points. First, when the environment supports independence, decision-making, and control for residents in memory care, they respond. The staff created a "cognitive ramp" to assist and enable their residents to act independently. This approach produced cooperative activity among residents, enhancing the development of interpersonal relationships. In addition, such environments support better health for residents. When older adults do not drink enough fluids, it is easier for them to contract urinary tract infections. When persons with dementia contract such an infection, it is common for them to become delirious, and often combative. Thus, by increasing independence, enhancing cooperation (such as in collectively deciding what fruits to put into the water and preparing them), increasing hydration, and thus reducing infections, a more peaceful environment is created both for residents and staff members.

Many memory care residences have gardens and/or landscaped areas. Ideally, these should be used by residents on a regular basis, as exposure to outdoor environments is good for residents (and anyone) both physically and mentally. However, in many instances, these environmental elements are not used. Again, giving residents "permission" to use elements of the environment is a method of empowering persons with dementia. Signs such as "Please come into the garden" or "Please enjoy the garden" may be crucial for residents to decide to go outside. In a similar way, signs in libraries or reading nooks should be posted, such as "Please take a book to read." Signs such as these can be accompanied by posters of older adults walking in gardens or reading books. Programmed activities using the environment, such as gardening (with raised beds that accommodate persons in walkers or wheelchairs) or reading clubs meeting on a regular basis in the library, increase the likelihood that environmental elements will be used. Ultimately, of course, you would want residents to be in charge of helping maintain the gardens and libraries. When residents view gardens, libraries, etc. as "theirs," they are more likely to use them and maintain them.

Other environmental characteristics, such as natural light and "non-institutional" overall features, are important as well. Elsewhere, we have described the use of input from a variety of different perspectives when designing such physical environments, including: universal design principles, geriatrics, dementia, disabilities research, the Montessori Method and its prepared environment, neuropsychological rehabilitation, human factors, and the role of the social environment (Camp *et al.* 2017). The following are a few examples from these areas, with an emphasis on the peace process. For more information on this topic (and any others in this book), please contact the authors using the contact details in Appendix 5.

Universal design principles support the creation of environments that accommodate as wide a variety of individuals as possible. For example, if there are residents with dementia who have a first language other than English, then signage in multiple languages should be a key feature in the environment. If you ever have been in a foreign country where the signs were not in your language and the people around you did not speak your language, you can understand how frustrating and frightening it can be to try to navigate, find out what is going on, find a place to eat, etc., under such conditions. Given that persons with dementia may revert to first languages as dementia progresses, the lack of understanding of signage and spoken language in their environments can lead to breakdowns in communication and conflict. Even for staff who speak English but not as their first language, seeing signage in their own tongues makes a difference. This little thing sends a powerful message about an environment that nurtures respect, dignity, and equality.

In addition, it encourages the use of multiple languages among residents and staff members. As we mentioned earlier, it is possible for persons with dementia to begin to learn words in a new language. When residents can greet one another in multiple languages, and when residents display a desire to learn words in languages spoken by other residents or staff members, an opportunity to nourish and encourage empathy presents itself. "Word of the Day" posters with words (and pronunciation guides) in different languages can encourage this practice. Ideally, the words and phrases to be learned would be chosen by the memory care residents, who would focus on communicating thoughts important to them (Antenucci *et al.* 2001).

Regarding geriatrics, it is critical that signage can be read by all or most of the residents. This involves ensuring that the print is large enough, that the font used does not involve thin or ornate lines (e.g. a sans serif font, such as Arial), that the contrast between printing and background is good (e.g. black print on white or pastel background), and that icons used in conjunction with print are both visible and comprehensible to residents. A drawing of a toilet may look like a hat to a person with dementia, but a "WC" or "Toilet" sign is unambiguous and a more effective environmental cue. Signage may need to be placed at multiple levels of height, to accommodate persons who are walking and who are in wheelchairs. A very simple but effective strategy is to present signage, icons, or any other environmental elements to residents with dementia and simply ask them to tell you what the elements say or mean. If a resident says that the icon you see as a toilet is a hat, there may be a reason why the resident does not go into that room if they need to urinate. Instead, they may search for a toilet, often in someone else's room.

Many conflicts arise in residential memory care because residents go into other residents' rooms. Have you ever put your key into the wrong room at a hotel? This often happens, and it is not because you have dementia. In many hotels, as is the case in many memory care residences, rooms look very similar. Have you ever forgotten your room number in a hotel? If you travel often, this can become commonplace. Imagine that you have dementia and are trying to remember your room number. Therefore, it is important to have landmarks for routes within a residence and multiple personalized cues at doorways and in the rooms of residents, to enable them both to find and recognize their own rooms *and* to recognize which rooms are not theirs. In addition, it is important for staff members to give residents practice in recognizing landmarks on routes and personalized cues. This is where neuropsychological rehabilitation comes into play. Just because signage or other cues have been placed in the environment does not mean that these elements will be used automatically and without error. It is the role of staff to enable residents in memory care to learn, in this case to learn to recognize and use signage, personalized environmental elements, etc., which requires practice. Thus, as always, the physical environment and social environment in memory care must work in concert to be effective in creating peaceful communities.

A resident in memory care had difficulty standing up straight, and so walked with a distinct stoop. She was reportedly having difficulty finding her own room, as well as being in the habit of entering other residents' rooms. Cameron invited her to show off her room. He led her to her doorway and asked, "Whose room is this?" She did not know, even though her name was on the door. However, since her name was at eye level for a person standing up straight, she could not see it. Guided into her room, the resident saw the quilt on her bed and said, "That's mine. This is my room." It was suggested that her name and a photo of her quilt be put in the entranceway to her room where she normally would look, given her posture, *and* that staff members give her practice looking at these cues and asking her what they signified.

A resident in one memory care setting, as she went to her seat at lunch, would use her cane to strike the legs of other residents seated along her path to her chair. The theory was that the woman assumed that other residents were invading her personal space, and that she needed to fend them off. This woman had advanced dementia, and so "reasoning" with her did not seem to help the situation. Instead, the staff created an ornate place mat and a beautiful tent card with the woman's name on it (she still could recognize her name) on a table with a chair at the other side of the room. Its location was at the beginning of her original line of march. This environmental modification, which made the new location more "attractive" in every sense of the word, curtailed her journey to find a seat for lunch and reduced the tension that had been associated with her at meals.

THE PEACE CORNER

An environmental element in many Montessori classrooms is a "peace corner." This is not to be confused with a tranquility room or a meditation site. These elements also can be part of a peaceful environment—a place where an individual can go to get away from the world and focus inward. The peace corner, on the other hand, is a "neutral corner," so to speak, where residents go with a mediator (and eventually without one) to settle differences. Here, as we have described previously, the rules for discussion are posted, and other environmental elements such as a talking stick are prominent. This is the location where residents can go to settle disagreements. The space does not have to be large (and, actually, should not be large)—just a table and chairs and the peace items. But having the peace corner labeled as such in the environment makes a statement about the values of the community.

In ancient Athens, the laws of the city were carved in marble and placed in the marketplace. It was done so that citizens could not say that they did not know about a law they had broken. In a similar way, it is important for the rules of any community to be posted and available for all to see. In addition, it helps to have "rules for visitors" developed by memory care residents. For example, in Helen's Place, these rules also are displayed prominently. The rules, provided to persons who plan to visit, include items such as the following:

- No tours during meals, though it is okay to come during programs. (This rule was made because residents decided that they did not like to be "looked at" while eating.)

- No profanity or swearing.

- Do not put your feet on the furniture.

- Please see a member of the Visitors' Committee to assist with your tour.

Note how these rules reflect the values and attitudes of persons who consider the place they live to be their home. For example, they do not condone profanity or swearing among themselves, and they do not want these behaviors brought in by visitors. Also note that asking visitors not to put their feet on the furniture reflects a pride of ownership and a sense that this place is the residents' home.

One cause of disturbance often seen in memory care is residents at the (usually locked) door of the residence saying that they want to go home. Encounters with residents in this situation can be very disruptive for staff members and other residents. The usual approach staff members are trained to implement is to try to distract the residents. However, this is only a temporary fix and does not address the cause of the behavior. The long-term fix is to create an environment that residents consider to be their home—a resident-driven community. When you are living at home, you do not need to leave to go home.

PEACEFUL COLORS

Often, we are asked about the best colors for memory care. Of course, colors such as bright red generally are not used in residential settings (or in the homes of individuals, with or without dementia). However, the question itself misses an important point. Once we were asked by a designer in Europe to describe the best color for a bedroom for a person with dementia. The person asking the question was a woman about 30 years old. Our response was, "What is the best color for a bedroom for all 30-year-old women? You are among the group of all women who are 30, so what is the best color for you and every other 30-year-old woman?" Our question proved to be disconcerting to the designer, but we followed up with the comment that if there was no one color for all 30-year-old women, there is no one color for all persons with dementia. We then said that she had asked the wrong question, and that instead her job should be to find a palette of acceptable colors from which each resident could choose their room's color, and a system to allow the color to be changed when another resident moved into the room (or the original resident changed his or her mind).

Thus, the environment for memory care must be capable of reflecting the personal tastes and preferences of its residents (since it is, after all, *their* home). In addition, the environment must be flexible to accommodate changes over time, given that residents will change over time and that new residents coming into the community will shape it in new ways.

CHAPTER 8

EXERCISES

WALKING AS A METHOD OF CONFLICT RESOLUTION

Another approach to conflict resolution can involve having the persons in conflict walk with each other. Webb, Rossignac-Milon and Higgins (2017) point out that there are many words and phrases associated both with conflict and with conflict resolution, such as "becoming stuck," "getting past," "moving forward," "standing one's ground," etc. They discuss many advantages of persons walking together, including the idea that walking helps us be more creative and flexible in our thinking. It can lower stress and increase positive emotions. Doing this together with another person, especially walking in synchrony side-by-side, may help people literally see things in the same way. They note that walking usually does not require much conscious effort, and can free the mind to think in more constructive ways. It is a novel approach to an old idea. As a couple, we often take a walk around the block when we want to try to solve a difficult problem, or at least think about the issues involved. It helps keep us on the same page, and seems to let us get to agreement more quickly and with less stress than sitting down at a table and just talking.

Of course, this approach may need to be modified for work with older populations and/or those with mobility challenges. Exercising on stationary bikes or pedal machines, moving together in wheelchairs, etc., could be tried. One thing to remember is that if the exercise is too strenuous it may impede the ability to think or let the mind move freely in constructive ways.

THE THANKING CIRCLE

A useful and effective activity to promote peace and empathy is the thanking circle (Malone *et al.* 2014). Residents sit in a circle and take turns giving thanks for an action, attribute, or something that was done by another resident. Participation always is voluntary, but seeing other residents offer thanks for a smile or a kindness performed by another can encourage quiet residents to watch and eventually also contribute (especially if they are the recipient of a thank you). The entire process is one that encourages residents to see the good in each other, while also emphasizing that positive behaviors are valued and expected as part of the community's culture.

This is an activity that should become a customary practice within a community and conducted on a regular (such as weekly) basis. Ideally, residents should help create the routine of the activity, such as choosing a song to sing or listen to for the opening part of the activity, choosing a poem or inspirational text to read aloud together for the closing of the activity, etc. Given that these residents have memory impairments, it helps to write down the "thank you" statements (such as "I want to thank Jane for always being so happy in the morning. It's contagious") on a flip chart or in some other manner so that they are easy to see. Also, lyrics for songs and words for poems or inspirational texts should be printed out (large print, sans serif font) so that residents do not necessarily have to remember the words.

READING GROUP ACTIVITIES

Another group activity that promotes empathy involves reading groups. For example, Reading Roundtable™ stories are designed so that one resident reads a page aloud while the other group members follow along. Then, another resident reads the next page aloud, and so on. During the reading of the stories and afterwards, questions for discussion are asked. Even if a person has trouble reading or is blind, the person can still listen and take part in the discussions. For example, there is a story from the Old Testament/Torah regarding Joseph and his coat of many colors. His brothers believed that he was the favorite of their father, became jealous of him, and sold him into slavery. It is a story of family disputes, powerful emotions, forgiveness and reconciliation. Reading and discussing stories about the need to forgive, settling differences amicably, etc., provides another opportunity to emphasize these ideas and to create expectations of mutual respect and peaceful resolutions of conflict within the community.

Touchstones® discussions

The materials in Touchstones® stories are designed to promote acceptance of differences of opinion. A short (usually one to one-and-a-half pages) story is read aloud, and all members of the group also have a written copy of it to follow along. A series of discussion questions follows the reading. For example, one story describes a discussion between Hector, the leader of the Trojan army during the war between the Trojans and the Greeks, and his wife, Andromache. At this point in the war, the greatest fighter for the Greeks, Achilles, has become angry with the leader of the Greek forces and has decided not to fight. Hector sees this as a chance to drive the Greeks back to their ships and win an ultimate victory. Andromache advises her husband to stay within the city and defend its walls. She reminds him that Achilles could change his mind, and that several of Hector's relatives already have been killed. She begs him not to leave the city to fight, and tells him that she does not want to become a widow or for Hector's child to become an orphan. Hector says that his men need for him to be a battle leader, and that he should not miss an opportunity to end the war. The discussion then centers around the question of whether or not Hector should follow the advice of his wife. Note that there is not a "right" answer to this question. Different options each have their merits and deficiencies. The point of the discussion is to learn to listen to opinions that differ from yours and to respect persons who do not agree with your way of thinking. Information about Touchstones® is found in Appendix 5. We currently are working with this organization to formulate these materials for use by persons with dementia, as well as developing the procedures to enable persons with dementia to lead these discussions.

OTHER "THINKING" ACTIVITIES

These are a few examples of "thinking" activities for persons with dementia. Just because persons have difficulty remembering more recent events does not mean that they are incapable of reasoning, discussing, or learning (as we mentioned in Chapter 3). There are many other types of activities that can generate discussion, such as reading advice column queries and then asking group members what advice they would give, listening to cases brought to court and then letting group members reach a verdict, etc. The common theme in these activities is that they always should have ground rules to ensure respectful listening and discussion, and these rules should be printed and visible to group members during discussions.

Again, ideally, these rules should be created and mutually agreed upon by residents. In addition, staff members should work to enable group activities to be as autonomous as possible, with members of the group becoming responsible for leading the activities, reminding members of the rules of conduct for the group, etc. Thus, these activities become ways of both forming community among residents as well as creating the culture of the community.

ALTRUISM AND CHARITABLE ACTIVITIES

Finally, it is important to enable residents to decide how they would like to contribute to the outside world and help other people who are in need (Camp, 2017; Camp *et al.* 2017). Having a bake sale or book sale to raise money for a school or charitable organization, collecting funds for victims of disasters, reading or teaching life skills to children, etc. are among the ways persons with dementia can give of themselves. As always, decisions should be made by residents, and all residents should be given an opportunity to contribute in whatever way they can. Even persons with advanced dementia may be able to shred old newspapers to make bedding for puppies in an animal shelter. Documenting these activities and the thanks received for them allows residents to see the results of their work in a way that circumvents memory deficits and encourages empathy and compassion.

CHAPTER 9

SUMMARY AND MOVING INTO THE FUTURE

Readers of this book will have realized by now that we are describing a way of living—one that must be lived every day. To begin to put these ideas and procedures into practice is to start a lifelong journey towards creating a more person-centered world for persons with dementia. This is about giving life back to these persons and enriching your own. The way of life we give to persons with dementia now is the one we will inherit for ourselves.

As imperfect human beings we make mistakes, but it is good to remember that Maria Montessori said that she welcomed her mistakes. They occur when we are attempting to continue to learn, innovate, try new things, and keep going forward. Mistakes are not failures if we use them as feedback and continue to grow as persons. Sharing this way of thinking with others is a gift—one we can give to our residents and staff and anyone else working with persons with dementia. It is a gift we can give to anyone.

There also is a saying to remember: "If you've seen one person with dementia, you've seen one person with dementia." Individuals and communities have their own unique personalities, customs, habits, etc. Our job is to find the best methods, environments, and techniques for the specific persons and communities we serve. Of course, communities and individuals themselves change and evolve over time, and so we must be willing to continually adapt and evolve our approaches, as well. Some elements of peaceful living, such as core values, will remain constant. Some methods of integrating these values into everyday living may change. Such is the nature of life.

We have tried to provide resources to enable you to continue to learn and apply the core values of peaceful living, empathy, and conflict resolution. Even when using a single technique, such as practicing mindfulness, one continues to learn and grow and develop new procedures with practice. This, like Montessori education, is an open-ended learning experience.

When starting on a new journey it helps to have companions who support you and who help you along the way. If you are interested in getting in touch with like-minded individuals, sharing your experiences, and learning from each other, please do contact us.[1] We would love to create an organization of persons who share the goal of creating peaceful, resident-driven communities for persons with dementia.

We often have been told that these ideas are revolutionary. We agree. Galileo put the sun at the center of the universe, and said that the earth revolved around the sun. This was a revolutionary idea. When we put persons with dementia at the center of our thinking and behavior, when we revolve around them, we too are promoting a revolutionary idea. Linda once suggested that we should use the term "evolution" instead of "revolution" to describe this approach to dementia

1   You can get in touch through our website: www.cen4ard.com.

care, but a colleague from Perth, Australia, said that he prefers revolutions—because they are faster. Finally, we often are asked when and where this revolution will begin. Our answer is always the same—here and now. We invite you, here and now, to join this peaceful revolution.

BIBLIOGRAPHY

Antenucci, V. M., Camp, C. J., Sterns, H., Sterns, R. and Sterns, A. (2001) 'Overcoming Linguistic and Cultural Barriers: Lessons from Long-Term Care Settings.' In K. H. Namazi and P. K. Chafetz (eds) *Assisted Living: Current Issues in Facility Management and Resident Care.* Westport, CT: Auburn House.

Bologna, S. M. and Camp, C. J. (1997) 'Covert versus overt self-recognition in late stage Alzheimer's disease.' *Journal of the International Neuropsychological Society 3,* 195–198.

Bourgeois, M., Camp, C., Rose, M., White, B., Malone, M., Carr, J. and Rovine, M. (2003) 'A comparison of training strategies to enhance use of external aids by persons with dementia.' *Journal of Communication Disorders 36,* 361–379.

Camp, C. J. (2006a) 'Montessori-Based Dementia Programming™ in Long-Term Care: A Case Study of Disseminating an Intervention for Persons with Dementia.' In R. C. Intrieri and L. Hyer (eds) *Clinical Applied Gerontological Interventions in Long-Term Care.* New York: Springer.

Camp, C. J. (2006b) 'Spaced Retrieval: A Case Study in Dissemination of a Cognitive Intervention for Persons with Dementia.' In D. Koltai Attix and K. A. Welsch-Bohmner (eds) *Geriatric Neuropsychological Assessment and Intervention.* New York: The Guilford Press.

Camp, C. J. (2012) *Hiding the Stranger in the Mirror: A Detective's Manual for Solving Problems Associated with Alzheimer's Disease and Related Disorders.* Solon, OH: Center for Applied Research in Dementia.

Camp, C. J. (2013) 'The Montessori approach to dementia care.' *Australian Journal of Dementia Care 2,* 5, 10–11.

Camp, C. J. (2017) 'Flexibility in Persons with Dementia.' In J. Sinnott (ed.) *Identity Flexibility during Adulthood: Perspectives in Adult Development.* New York: Springer.

Camp, C. J., Antenucci, V. M., Schreckenberger, C. and Kotich, W. (2017) 'Memory care: Integrating the physical and social environments.' Annual Convention of the American Society on Aging, Chicago, IL. 20–24 March 2017.

Camp, C. J., Bird, M. J. and Cherry, K. E. (2000) 'Retrieval Strategies as a Rehabilitation Aid for Cognitive Loss in Pathological Aging.' In R. D. Hill, L. Bäckman and A. S. Neely (eds) *Cognitive Rehabilitation in Old Age.* New York: Oxford University Press.

Camp, C. J. and Nasser, E. H. (2003) 'Nonpharmacological Aspects of Agitation and Behavioral Disorders in Dementia: Assessment, Intervention, and Challenges to Providing Care.' In P. A. Lichtenberg, D. L. Murman and A. M. Mellow (eds) *Handbook of Dementia: Psychological, Neurological, and Psychiatric Perspectives.* New York: John Wiley & Sons.

Camp, C. J. and Skrajner, M. J. (2016) 'Direct Cognitive Therapy Techniques for Persons with Dementia and Related Cognitive Disorders.' In P. R. Johnson (ed.) *A Clinician's Guide to Successful Evaluation and Treatment of Dementia.* Gaylord, MI: Northern Speech Services.

Camp, C. J., Antenucci, V. M., Roberts, A., Fickenscher, T., Erkes, J. and Neal, T. (2017) 'The Montessori Method applied to persons with dementia: An international perspective.' *Montessori Life 29,* 41–47.

Center for Applied Research in Dementia (n.d.) *Montessori Inspired Lifestyle® Pledge.* Accessed on 6 November 2017 at https://www.cen4ard.com/index.php?option=com_content&view=article&id=80&Itemid=605.

Cohen-Mansfield, J. (2015) 'Behavioural and Psychological Symptoms of Dementia.' In P. A. Lichtenberg and B. T. Mast (editors-in-chief) *APA Handbook of Clinical Geropsychology. 2. Assessment, Treatment, and Issues of Later Life.* Washington, D.C.: American Psychological Association.

Drew, N. (1991) *The Peaceful Classroom in Action.* Torrance, CA: Jalmar Press.

Hühnel, I., Fölster, M., Werheid, K. and Hess, U. (2014) 'Empathic reactions of younger and older adults: No age-related decline in affective responding.' *Journal of Experimental Social Psychology 50,* 136–143.

Kitwood, T. (1997) *Dementia Reconsidered: The Person Comes First.* Maidenhead: Open University Press.

Langer, E. J. (2014) *Mindfulness: 25th Anniversary Edition*. Philadelphia, PA: De Capo Press.

Lillard, A. S. (2011) 'Mindfulness practices in education: Montessori's approach.' *Mindfulness 2*, 78–85.

Malone, M. L., Skrajner, M. J., Camp, C. J. and Zgola, J. M. (2014) 'Disseminating a Philosophy of Care: Translating the Work of Jitka Zgola.' In J. Duvvuru, J. M. Kalavar, A. M. Khan and P. S. Liebig (eds) *Global Ageing: Care Concerns and Special Perspectives*. New Delhi, India: Kanishka Publishers.

Mast, B. T., Shouse, J. and Camp, C. J. (2015) 'Person-Centered Assessment and Intervention for People with Dementia.' In P. A. Lichtenberg and B. T. Mast (editors-in-chief) *APA Handbook of Clinical Geropsychology. 2. Assessment, Treatment, and Issues of Later Life*. Washington, D.C.: American Psychological Association.

Merriam-Webster (2017) *Peace*. Accessed on 16 October 2017 at www.merriam-webster.com/dictionary/peace.

Montessori, M. (1971) *Peace and Education: 5th Edition*. Adyar, Madras 20, India: Theosophical Publishing House.

Skrajner, M. J., Haberman, J. L., Camp, C. J., Tusick, M., Frentiu, C. and Gorzelle, G. (2014) 'Effects of using nursing home residents to serve as group activity leaders: Lessons learned from the RAP Project.' *Dementia 13*, 2, 274–285.

van der Ploeg, E. S., Eppingstall, B., Camp, C. J., Runci, S. J., Taffe, J. and O'Connor, D. W. (2013) 'A randomized cross-over trial to study the effect of personalized, one-to-one interaction using Montessori-based activities on agitation, affect and engagement in nursing home residents with dementia.' *International Psychogeriatrics 25*, 565–575.

Webb, C. E., Rossignac-Milon, M. and Higgins, E. T. (2017) 'Stepping forward together: Could walking facilitate interpersonal conflict resolution?' *American Psychologist 72*, 374–385.

Wolf, C. and Serpa, J. G. (2014) *A Clinician's Guide to Teaching Mindfulness*. Oakland, CA: New Harbinger Publications, Inc.

PEACE PLEDGES

Here are some places to find examples of peace pledges:

www.ngl.org/pledge-of-peace.html

www.kidsforpeaceglobal.org

More examples can be found through internet searches. However, of course, the best peace pledge is the one created by residents themselves.

GUIDELINES FOR A PEACEFUL COMMUNITY

Here are some school-based references and examples of guidelines for a peaceful community:

> https://anconaschool.org/school-guidelines/
> peaceful-learning-community

> http://peacefulschoolsinternational.org/wp-
> content/uploads/USIP-Guide-April-2012.pdf

> www2.peacefirst.org/digitalactivitycenter/system/
> files/activities/files/classroom_contract_tipsheet.pdf

The questions in this last reference, such as: "How would you like to be treated in this community?" and "What would make you feel safe?" can be used to help guide discussion among residents to create their own guidelines.

Here is a resource for creating a sense of community:

> www.thecommunitymanager.com/2013/11/19/
> the-psychology-of-communities-4-factors-
> that-create-a-sense-of-community

FAIR FIGHTING

Here are useful resources that provide more information regarding fair fighting:

https://happylists.wordpress.com/2008/08/01/37-rules-to-fighting-fair

www.cmhc.utexas.edu/fightingfair.html

MINDFULNESS

Here are resources for using mindfulness with persons with dementia:

www.carewatch.co.uk/blog/using-mindfulness-with-dementia/4739

www.wihealthyaging.org/_data/files/C4._Med_Dem_Literature_Reivew.pdf

Resources for mindfulness use by caregivers:

www.alz.org/mnnd/documents/Session_310_Handout1.pdf

AARP Meditations for Caregivers: Practical, Emotional, and Spiritual Support for You and Your Family by Barry J. Jacobs and Julia L. Mayer (2016) Boston, MA: Da Capo Lifelong Books [This is available at Amazon.com]

Excellent general resources include:

A Clinician's Guide to Teaching Mindfulness by Christiane Wolf and J. Greg Serpa (2015) Oakland, CA: New Harbinger Publications.

www.positivepsychologyprogram.
com/mindfulness-meditation

Here is a site with a number of mindfulness activities for children that can be modified to work with adults with dementia:

www.positivepsychologyprogram.com/
mindfulness-for-children-kids-activities

Finally, here is an example of the way mindfulness has been a component of Montessori education from its inception:

www.faculty.virginia.edu/ASLillard/
PDFs/Lillard%20(2011).pdf

GENERAL RESOURCES

CONFLICT RESOLUTION

Here are some references on **training for, and managing, conflict resolution**:

http://ctb.ku.edu/en/table-of-contents/
implement/provide-information-enhance-
skills/conflict-resolution/main

Hiding the Stranger in the Mirror, mentioned in the text, is in paperback or ebook and available at our website: www.cen4ard.com. We also can help provide you with German, Italian, French or Spanish translations of the text. More languages will be available soon.

The **FLIP-IT** model for dealing with challenging behaviors in children also can be modified to work with older adults with dementia. Here is its website: www.centerforresilientchildren.org/flip-it

Montessori and Peace: Here is a downloadable resource written by Maria Montessori herself. Reading it, you can understand why she was nominated for the Nobel Peace

Prize three times: https://ia800206.us.archive.org/20/items/Peace_And_Education_/peace_and_education__text.pdf

Here is a resource guide for creating a Montessori peace corner. Again, it is written with a school setting in mind, but the ideas in it can be translated into dementia residential settings very easily: www.montessorirocks.org/montessori-how-to-peace-corner-calming-jar

Bathing/Mouth Care without a Battle are excellent resources for caregivers who wish to reduce conflict and agitation when delivering personal care for these two highly personal and sensitive tasks:

Bathing Without a Battle: www.bathingwithoutabattle.unc.edu

Bathing Without a Battle: Personal Care of Individuals with Dementia edited by Ann Louise Barrick, PhD., Joanne Rader, Beverly Hoeffer, Philip D. Sloane (2001) New York: Springer Publishing Company. Available at https://books.google.com/books?hl=en&lr=&id=BQgcaZJe874C&oi=   fnd&pg=PP11&dq=bathing+without+battle&ots =QZDQFu5Pub &sig=YPLkoXAiIC7Egpmq cGxOsGwj dtA#v=onepage &q=bathing%20without%20battle&f= false

Mouth Care without a Battle: www.mouthcarewithoutabattle.org

SOSS

Here are some resources elaborating the SOSS approach. More are available through searching the internet:

www.chuckdawson.com/Amygdala%20Hijack2.pdf

www.ezinearticles.com/?If-Youre-Triggered,-Send-an-SOS(S)&id=2581404

www.dhhr.wv.gov/healthprep/about/archives/Documents/VERNAL%20-%20Emotional%20Intelligence.pdf

TOUCHSTONES®

Here is the Touchstones® website: www.touchstones.org

SPACED-RETRIEVAL

Tactus Therapy describes spaced-retrieval in a page on their website: www.tactustherapy.com/spaced-retrieval-training-memory

They also have a downloadable app for using spaced-retrieval that is not very expensive.

For more extensive training on the use of spaced-retrieval, an online course on the topic can be found at the website of Northern Speech Services: www.northernspeech.com/brain-injury-mild-traumatic/spaced-retrieval-a-therapy-technique-for-improving-memory-for-task-completion-addresses-communication-and-swallowing

Other resources, or publications on mindfulness, can be obtained by visiting our website and contacting us:

Center for Applied Research in Dementia
34194 Aurora Road #182
Solon, OH 44132
Cameron@cen4ard.com
www.cen4ard.com

INDEX

Adaptive Interaction and Dementia
How to Communicate without Speech

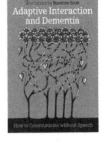

Dr Maggie Ellis and Professor Arlene Astell
Illustrated by Suzanne Scott

Paperback: £19.99 / $26.95
ISBN: 978 1 78592 197 1
eISBN: 978 1 78450 471 7

192 pages

This guide to Adaptive Interaction explains how to assess the communication repertoires of people with dementia who can no longer speak, and offers practical interventions for those who wish to interact with them.

Outlining the challenges faced by people living with advanced dementia, this book shows how to relieve the strain on relationships between them, their families, and professional caregivers through better, person-centred communication. It includes communication assessment tools and guidance on how to build on the communication repertoire of the individual with dementia using nonverbal means including imitation, facial expressions, sounds, movement, eye gaze and touch. With accessible evidence and case studies based on the authors' research, *Adaptive Interaction* can be used as the basis for developing interactions without words with people living with dementia.

Dr Maggie Ellis is Lecturer at the School of Psychology & Neuroscience, University of St Andrews, UK. **Arlene Astell** is Professor at the School of Psychology & Clinical Language Sciences, University of Reading, UK and at the Department of Occupational Sciences & Occupational Therapy, University of Toronto, Canada.

Understanding Behaviour in Dementia that Challenges, Second Edition
A Guide to Assessment and Treatment
Ian Andrew James and Louisa Jackman

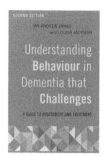

Paperback: £25.00 / $35.00
ISBN: 978 1 78592 264 0
eISBN: 978 1 78450 551 6

320 pages

The innovative Newcastle Challenging Behaviour Model for dementia care has recently been updated, leading to new advances in the field. This revised second edition guide to assessment and treatment of behaviours that challenge associated with dementia includes these latest developments along with new sections on what have traditionally been considered controversial topics.

The new chapters cover issues including:
- End of life care
- Use of therapeutic dolls
- Lies and deception
- Physical restraint during personal care
- Racism towards care staff

With a particular emphasis on non-pharmacological approaches, this book details the range of behaviours common in individuals with dementia, along with the most effective assessment and treatment techniques for health care professionals.

Ian Andrew James is Challenging Behaviour Trust Lead for Older People and Consultant Clinical Psychologist in Northumberland Tyne and Wear NHS Trust. Ian is also an Honorary Professor at Bradford University.

Dr Louisa Jackman worked in Older People's Psychological Services for 13 years until recently moving to work in neuropsychology. She now works with people with Acquired Brain Injury in Northumberland, Tyne & Wear NHS Trust.